poemspartum

poemspartum: pregnancy, postpartum, motherhood, seasons (growth)
Copyright © 2024 by Kassondra Mangione
All rights reserved. No part of this book may be reproduced, scanned, or distributed in any printed or electronic form without permission.
FIRST EDITION
Artwork by Hannah Hawthorne
Printed in the United States of America
ISBN: 9798325848186

poemspartum

pregnancy, postpartum, motherhood, seasons (growth)

kassondra mangione

to my girls, who are the wind in my sails, and to my
husband, who is my anchor in every storm.

and to all the mothers, parents, and readers who will take
something from this book:
i see you. i hear you. you are loved.

thus emerged a poet

my friend said that
postpartum unveiled a secret vault
hidden behind vines and tangles of uncertainty
and when it opened
a poet emerged.
she was uncertain at first
blinking blindly in the sunlight
but she was filled to the brim
and ready to pour out her soul
so that other mothers
feeling grief
feeling alone
feeling too much
but never enough
could trace their fingers
over the familiar words
and feel at home.

pregnancy

sore

weaving through the home maintenance aisles
i thought i felt
a twinge in my breasts
an ache like a weight
hot and heavy.

could it be?
i smiled to myself
flitting my fingers over paint brush bristles
eyeing the pink and blue swatches
                                        dreaming.

my husband whistled one aisle over
unaware that finding the best light fixture
would be the least of his worries very soon.

double line

i sit on my bed and stare at the closed bathroom door
my phone timer counting down
wishing time would stand still and yet

                                        speed up!

i couldn't take another month of rejection.

i couldn't take another month
of what did i do wrongs
of dipping sticks
of avoiding questions
of double tapping other pregnancy announcements
of wondering when my time would come.

the timer rings
and i go in and see

a double line.

seasick

i've been on a boat a few times.
i grew up on the shore, after all.

i envision the waves crashing
the boat rocking
and me clutching the sides
my stomach turning
acid reaching the top of my throat
the relief never coming

… i feel like i am on a boat.

pillows

there's one for my head
and one for my upper back
and one for my knees
and one for my swelling ankles:
four pillows on our queen-sized bed.

plus three cats
plus insomnia
plus heartburn
plus crippling fear that leaves me gasping in the night.

add in a snoring husband
and you have a very tired and very awake pregnant woman.

breech

'she won't turn,' they said.
turn … where?

her head is in my ribs
(which explained the heartburn)
(and the excruciating pain)

so my options were to
        let it be
or
go to the hospital at 37 weeks
get a spinal tap
and feel immense pressure
as they try to push my baby head down
for a 'normal' birth.

i could have some bleeding
she could go into distress
i could go into early labor.

in the end,
i chose to let it be.

'the last time i am in control,' i said.

to my husband

i chose you for many reasons:
for your kind eyes
that crinkle when you smile.
for your laugh
and silliness
that only i get to see.

but i also chose you
because i knew
that during those late, scary nights
you'd wipe the tears
as i held new life in my arms.

because i knew
that you would step in
when i was at my lowest
no complaints
no judgment
just unconditional love.

because i knew
you'd roll up your sleeves
and you'd do the work
the real shit
you'd give one hundred percent
every day
for us.

and i chose you
because you see me as an equal
in partnership
in domesticity
in marriage
in parenthood.

let's do this all over again, huh?

grows

how it is possible
that
my heart has room
for one more baby?

it's already filled to the brim
with inexplicable and unmeasurable
adoration
joy
love.

so much
that i am close to
        bursting
every day.

how will i find the space
for this new life
growing in my belly?

daughters

it's another girl, they said,
and i immediately thought of fire.

i thought of clenched fists and a lifetime of what-ifs
i thought of nervous glances and not taking chances.

i thought of a house filled with frilly dresses
of tights and messes

i thought of emotions
                        overflowing …

of dollhouses and tea parties
of clothing and fashion trends
of teasing and bullying
precious friendships lost
then true sisterhoods made.

i thought of growing up before you should.
i thought of a lot of things.

like how maybe boys would have been easier …
and how hard it is to be a woman.

i thought about body autonomy
about birth control
about marriage equality
about silencing and pay gaps
about the male gaze.

but then i thought about me
about *me* raising strong women
and how i will teach them that
"no."
is a complete sentence.

i will teach them how to speak their mind
i will teach them to be fearless
i will teach them to be an ally.

i will teach them
to read
to think
to dream
to achieve
to explore
to climb rocks and jump and play
to inspire.

i will teach them
how to be an ember
that sets the world on fire.

wake before the sky

sometimes
i will wake before the sky opens its eyes.

i will tiptoe past my snoring husband
soundlessly step down the hall
carefully avoid the creaky floorboards
and head
       down
              the
                      groaning
                                stairs
of my new england home

to have a quiet morning by myself.

the only sounds
are the larks crooning
and the coffee brewing
to help fuel a tired mother
as she grows another life.

a tired mother
trying to shut out the noise
of to-do lists and errands
of 'i shoulds' and 'i needs.'

a tired mother
trying to have a moment
to silently
i n h a l e
e x h a l e
to be.
to peacefully start her day.

mommy

your shout pierces the night
and i wake with a
                          jolt!

i carefully get out of bed
holding my swollen belly
and silently shuffle to your room.

it still smells like bath time.
of oranges and cream
of giggles and stolen smooches
of story time and toothpaste.

you stand in your crib
hair tussled and eyes red
and i pick you up
under your outstretched arms
and kiss away those salty tears
hush the fears
and rock in our favorite chair.

you don't
quite fit
like you used to

your body
splayed
over my
round tummy

you reach
for my hair
and give small tugs

as we rock
in the safe silence.

your baby sister
keeping rhythm
with her
kicks and twirls

and i think
can life
get any better
than this?

last night

as i was tossing and turning in bed
like a large rotisserie chicken
i had a great idea for a poem.

but like every thought i have lately
it came and went
like a tiny feather
coasting on a cool breeze.

so, you'll have to settle for this one,
dear reader,
and the poems that have come before it.

to times when my eyes weren't as heavy
and my words found their home.

midnight cheerios

is there anything better
than a bowl of honey nut cheerios
at midnight?

'sleeping, probably,'
thinks the pregnant woman
as she desperately
waits
for reprieve.

worries

she has so many worries.

she wears them like chains
hanging from her neck.
pinning her ankles down to the earth.

she just wants to
                       float
to
  d r i f t
                       off to sleep.

but the flurry of thoughts
fears
restlessness
keeps her eyes peeled open.

her
heart
races

her chest aches
she feels like she is
       breaking.

… when she's already come undone.

she just wants to sleep.

but her back, her hips, her spine, her legs
throb
under the weight
of the baby that grows in her belly.

but also under the weight
of 'what ifs'
and of 'how will she' … ?

her mind and body
just won't quit
but she needs to rest
to make it all happen tomorrow.

so, she puts down her pen
and starts the journey back upstairs
to try again.

eva james

you are almost here,
our sweet little eva james.
i am counting down
the minutes – the days –
until i get to stare at your sweet, sleeping face.

i am counting down the days

until the restless nights
when i peek in your bassinet
to watch the gentle rise and fall of your chest.

until the swollen breasts
and when the angry pink scar, once healed
is reopened to heal again.

until i see your big sister
my beautiful, growing, gentle girl
give you a hug and kiss.

until the quiet mornings
when the sun is still abed
but we are up
rocking
and soaking in the moments
just you and me.

i am counting down the days
until you are home
until we are complete.

postpartum

feb. 3, my nora lee

feb. 3 was the day i was born too.
when i became a mother forever.

it was the day i held life
the day that i saw you and went:
'oh, there you are.'

the day i realized you were the piece that was missing
the day i just stared and wondered
the day when i finally let out an exhale
and looked at my husband and fell in love with him
        all over again.
the day that i surprised myself
when i realized that i am invincible.

the day i felt free
the day i felt whole
was the day you came
oh, my girl, my nora lee,
happy birthday to you and me.

little blue pill

it's my favorite color
a tiffany blue.

this little pill
will serve as my crutch
to help me walk
a tiny cylindrical life vest to keep me
                a f l o a t.

a few days ago, i woke in the hospital room
and i didn't see you nearby
so the world

stopped.

i gasped
my vision blurred
my heart monitor beeped
my husband coaxed
as he showed me where you were.

'she's ok,' he said, holding you in his arms.
'she's here. she's safe.'

the nurses came in
to hush and soothe
wiping tears and snot
bringing ginger ale and ice chips.

the doctor came later
and holding my hands
        she listened.

and i wept
i shook
and she told me you would help.

i knew the anxiety was inevitable.
it lay dormant in my belly for months.
a pile of embers waiting to be stoked.
and then you came, and it caught flame.

i welcomed the panic
the emptied lungs
the dark thoughts
the sudden loneliness
the dread
like an old friend.

but i want to be free of it.

so, will you, little blue pill
dampen the flame?
help me inhale?
guide me to the lighthouse?

will you help me find her again?

the stranger

for nine months
i watched my body grow for you
i watched in awe
magic personified.

before, i saw a warrior
but now
i see a creature
with a sagging stomach
and stretch marks on my legs,
my arms,
      my breasts.
swollen ankles
and a red, angry scar.

'what about *me*?!'
i scream
'where did she go?
'and who is this stranger
covered in spit-up
and masked in guilt?
this isn't *me*.
i have a routine
order
      structure!'

i'm in there somewhere.

but for now,
i see a stranger.

sleepless nights

i can't say that people didn't warn me.

that i'd spend countless nights
staring at the ceiling
while my world
slept soundlessly around me.

that i'd watch her sleep
with my eyes peeled open
waiting for this perfect gift
to be snatched away from me.

yes, people mentioned the panic.
but they didn't mention the foul, sour taste of fear.
how it'd rise in my throat at any given moment.

and they didn't mention the mania.

the hitch of
        breath
my muffled sobs echoing from the steaming shower.

that i'd spend most of my waking moments
in those early months
battling the darkest thoughts.
the visions that i didn't dare to share
the fears i couldn't say out loud.

the insurmountable pain (and joy!) that i'd feel
now that you are here.
emotions so vast that my body could not take it.

all those sleepless nights.

letdown

a large bubble
close to b u r s t i n g
a tiny head brought to my breast.
then a sharp shooting sensation
like prickly heat.
here comes the
letdown
and then
silent suckling in a quiet, sleepy house
met with a mama's great relief.

tired

achy bones
fuzzy brain
mumble grumble

identity

i'm two different people, you see
trying to make it all work
in one body.

in one body that barely gets any sleep
in one body that doesn't have time to eat
or drink hot coffee.

in one body that is overworked
because i carry all the burdens.

i carry them on my shoulders
i carry them right at the base of my skull
and then transfer them to one hip
as i balance you on the other.

and when i catch a glimpse of myself in the mirror
i cackle
because why didn't my husband tell me
that my hair looked like bees swarmed through it
or that i had boogers on my shirt? (not mine …)

i want to be it all.

the fit mom
the healthy mom
the successful, working mom
the mom who writes.

but more importantly
i want to be a present mom
a loving mom
a patient mom.

i want to know how it is possible
to fit all of this
in one body.

in the body of
the same woman
who just realized
her shirt
has been inside out all day.

i just want, i wish

i just want to protect you
from the things that go bump in the night.

from the monsters under the bed
and from those that live inside my head.

i wish i could put an indestructible bubble
around your perfect, tiny body
to ward off anything that tries
to bruise
to scare
to scar.

i just want to turn off
the news
my anxious thoughts
my worries
my catastrophizing, maddening, uncontrollable brain.

you are too precious to be tainted.
already too smart for this world.
but still too innocent to realize
that not everyone will make you smile.

that one day
i will disappoint you.
that one day
your dreams will be crushed
somehow, some way.

i will just do my best
to control the things i can.
and protect you
as you grow.

hush

have you ever pointed out an insecurity in front of
coworkers
friends
family
because you feared they already thought it?

that instead of listening to your story
they saw the extra weight
clinging around your waist
because your baby
still nurses
and you have yet to 'bounce back'
to the old you?
do you think they even notice those things?

what about instead they are in awe of your intelligence?
or your bright eyes?
or your smile?
or your kind, good soul?

what if they are just happy to be around you?
to know you?
and have you here
in their little corner of the world?

so, my dear friend, try not to say it.

hush.

because they don't see it.
i certainly don't see it.

and please know
that you are worth more
than the little voice inside
telling you 'no.'

'the yellow wallpaper'

when i first read charlotte's story
i thought
'who does the woman really see within the yellow walls?'

i realize now that she saw me.
and my best friend.
and my mother.
and my grandmother.
and my great-grandmother.
and perhaps she sees you, too.

she watches as we try to claw ourselves out.
we are fighting for our lives.
our sanity.
one year, five years, thirty years, fifty years postpartum.

we are trying to escape
the thick coating of self-loathing
of hatred.
and we wonder
if we are indeed mad
or if instead
it's society
that's confined us to these walls.

trapped behind
the yellow wallpaper.

blushing cheeks

when my baby closes her eyes
and drifts off to sleep
i stay a while longer
just to stare.

i watch her eyelids flicker
her lips twitch
and listen as her breathing
slows to sleepy snores.

and i think about how much it hurts
to love someone this much.
so much
that the word 'love'
seems inadequate.

and my chest just swells
and i wonder if it's going to explode
and i breathe in your smell
softly brush your blushing cheeks
and whisper something sweet.

in a dark hospital room

i.

in a dark hospital room
a mother breathes
s l o w l y
eyes closed
listening to the beeps
and sounds
of the machines
that help her body heal.

ii.

in a dark hospital room
a mother weeps
as her husband carries away the milk
that she pumped from her breasts
the milk that they will save
for their newborn baby they left behind
along with her big sister
safe at home.

iii.

in a dark hospital room
a mother waits
for the next blood pressure reading
for the iron to stop dripping
for the compression boots to stop pumping
for the chest x-ray results
she wants to go home.

in a dark hospital room
a mother googles
even though she shouldn't.
she looks up 'postpartum preeclampsia'
that god-damned, rare, life-threatening condition

that took her away from her babies
one-week postpartum.

iv.

in a dark hospital room
a mother prays
for the first time in a long time.

she prays for good results.
she prays for a long, healthy life.
she prays to hear those soft, sweet breaths
from her sleeping girls.
she prays to feel those sticky, peanut-butter toddler fingers
caress her face as she carries her girl upstairs for bath time.

vi.

in a dark hospital room
a mother wants
to go home.

if i died tomorrow

if i died tomorrow
would they remember me?

'don't think that,' you say,
but can you blame me?

they are every part of me
they are my reason for *being*
but if i were to die tomorrow
you would have to tell them just how much
i loved my girls.

you would have to tell them
that i had a funny laugh
      and that little snort nora has is from me.
that i drank way too much coffee.
that i collected stickers.
that i loved to sing.

you would have to tell them
because they wouldn't remember me.

if i died tomorrow,
they would only have this poem
because they wouldn't have me.

'this is how i am healing today'

i whisper to myself
as i walk around my yard
with rosy, tear-stained cheeks
my feet crunching over the grass
breaking through the morning frost.

'this is how i am healing today,'
i murmur to the lilac tree
willing for a bud to show itself
so i know that there's hope for me too.

'this is how i am healing today,'
i say to the clouds
begging the sun
to warm us all
to melt away the cold
so i can plant my roots
deep into the earth
and begin again.

newborn snuggles

and sometimes newborn *struggles*?

yes, that too.
it's ok to experience both, yes?

i am nap trapped, and i am loving
her smell
her warmth
her staccato breath
her trust.

but i am also feeling
suffocated
unproductive
anxious
… under a magnifying glass.

how much do you want me to be, world?
so much that i believe i am never enough?

'just breathe,' i whisper,
'and try to enjoy this fleeting season.'

motherhood

when you're sick

when you're sick
i feel lost
      stuck
            paralyzed

with guilt.

because i can only do so much
to help take the pain away.

i wish i could take it myself.

that i could have the fever
the congestion
the rashes
the sweats and the terrors.

i would take it all
ten times over
to heal you
and see your smile again.

quiet nights

late at night
when my mind is alive
i lie in bed
close my eyes
and listen to the silence.

if i concentrate hard enough
i can hear your soft breathing in the other room
the slow, rhythmic breaths
of a safe baby
surrounded by her bears
and the sweet colors
of her nursery.

then i think about how earlier that night
when i asked for a hug and a kiss
you stuck your tongue out at me instead
and we both laughed.

then i smile
and fall asleep.

i'm sorry i yelled

i'm sorry i yelled
but i feel like i failed you
when i couldn't get you to calm down.

i'm sorry i yelled
when you were screaming during a work call.
it's not your fault
another kid got you sick
and daycare won't let you in.

i'm sorry i yelled
when you were just trying to tell me
that you are afraid of taking medicine
and you don't understand
that it will take away the pain.

i'm just so sorry i yelled
because i am really trying
to be a good mom.

hot coffee

i always underestimated
the irrevocable beauty
of drinking a steaming cup of coffee
on a sunday morning.

the memories flood in
of me flipping through a magazine
pausing to take sips from my ceramic mug
looking out the window
just me and my coffee.

i think about those times often
as i stand at the microwave
and wait
for my ice-cold coffee
to be reheated
for the third time
that morning.

... and a hot coffee haiku

a hot steaming mug
of coffee in the morning
is just a memory.

pant leg

oh, my pant leg
your favorite thing to tug.
except for my last nerve
as i get you another cracker
the one that you very kindly
screamed about wanting …

your sixth one this morning.

can i just have a minute

to myself?

        a minute?!

to think
to eat
to use the bathroom?

can i just have a minute
to write this poem?

to think about something other than
sunscreen
daycare pickups
bathing suits
fevers
butt cream?

can i just have a minute
to eat my lunch
without having to share?

can i just have a minute
to hop on the treadmill
to lose the weight
that still clings to my hips?

can i just have a minute
to schedule a hair appointment?
because if i don't do it right now
i am going to forget.

can i just have a minute
to read something other than
the little blue truck?

and no, my 3 a.m. google searches about your face rash does not count.

can i just have a minute
a minute to myself
to mindlessly scroll on my phone
and look at pictures of you?

today it finally rained

after what seemed like ages.

buckets of it
dripping
like a triumphant drumbeat
on my roof.

the ground's mouth
open wide
thirsty
drinking the moisture
it so desperately craved.

i thought about past rainy days
when i was 'baby-free'
lighting candles
fairy lights twinkling
in the cozy aesthetic of my home
a warm, hazy glow.

i thought about chai tea lattes
soup simmering on the stove
cats snoring on the sofa
peace and quiet
as i leafed through a good book
the smell of cinnamon and turmeric
and cold, wet earth.

today, my rainy day looks different.

it's filled with tantrums
and tripping over toys.

it's filled with rushed sips of lukewarm coffee
of hurried lunches and short tempers.
of nap time negotiations.
oh, how i miss those early days.

if i am honest, sometimes i yearn to taste
that independence again.
i dream of those quiet, rainy mornings.

but i know that when my hair turns gray
and my home is empty
i will find myself
sitting at my kitchen table
on a rainy day
listening to the raindrops
thinking
       wishing
              to trip over toys
              to scrape an uneaten lunch in the compost bin
              to quell a meltdown
              to put a sleepy child in her crib while she
              sings about the rain
              asking for it to come back another day.

a day to myself

'you can have the day to yourself,' he said.

so i decided to tend to my plants.

i snipped their
dead
      ends.

and i gave them some water to drink.

i fed them fresh compost so they can come back strong.

and i spoke to them
in sweet, nurturing whispers
complimenting their growth
admiring their blooms
appreciating their place
in this wide, wide world.
small
but significant to me.

when i was done, i smiled to myself.

              'always a mama …' i realized.

so i grabbed my book
an ice-cold drink
laid in my hammock
allowing its protective cradle
to rock me to sleep.

those first steps

you looked at me with those sly eyes that i love so much
and then suddenly
you pushed yourself up on your chubby legs
and took your first steps
your face triumphant
squealing with delight.

and i cried.

look at our girl go.
look at what she will become.

bath time

i really enjoy bath time
and its silence — interrupted
by soapy splashes
and echoey squeals
from a little girl
scrubbed clean
from the day's adventures.

scrubbed clean
from crusty, oatmeal-covered eyebrows
from dirty knees
and from sun-screened skin.

just a little girl
and her toys
and a tub filled with wonders.
and her smiling mama
who has lived
another perfect day.

a rhetorical question for a poet

as a poet
have you ever
found yourself in your busy day
saying: 'oh!
that would make a great poem.'

you try to squeeze the idea
inside your slippery, spongey mind
but it isn't so porous anymore
because of daycare pickups
and bedtimes
and gyno appointments
and upcoming maternity leave.

when the house is finally quiet
from its clanging dishes
and pattering footsteps
you sit down
open your notebook
and find
that the good idea
is gone
                        lost.

it got lost.
perhaps in the brambles of some bush.
or at the playground.

or did you leave it
on the pantry shelf
next to the jam?

or is it still at the supermarket
shouting:
'wait! come back!
you forgot about me … again!'

bunny

my daughter came home today
with a stuffed bunny
that was brown all over.

its white tail
was tattered from age
and its ribbons were shredded
from years of being grasped
by tiny hands.

my daughter carries it around
by its long ears
his body bouncing
as she tots around the room.

he sits next to her
and she plants kisses on his brown bunny nose
while she plays with her blocks
stacking them high to the sky.

the next day
we take bunny in the car to return him to daycare
and i learn that he belongs to the woman's daughter
who is now grown.

her daughter said my baby could keep it
because she's too old for it now.
too old to stroke its fur
and hold it tight in the night.
too old to give it kisses
on a colorful rug
next to a pile of blocks.

and i was sad
because one day
my baby will give the bunny away
to a little girl who needs it more.

tonight, i danced

with my mother and my grandmother
and my baby joined in.

we swayed in the living room
dancing
being silly
clapping to the music.

we laughed and sang and twirled
to jazz and classic rock
songs from my childhood
from the days when i was my daughter's size
watching my mother
dance with her mother
and grandmother.

i smiled and felt angry all at once
at the fragility and impermanence
of life.
how the world rips people from our grasp
until all that's left are memories
written down in poetic prose
with the purpose
to make that moment
last forever.

complete

i was so nervous
about bringing you into our little world.

but once i saw my nora
laugh big belly laughs
as she held you in her arms
i let out a giant exhale of relief
and said to myself
'now, we are complete.'

time to let go

if they were boys,
would you be around?

did you wish that we were boys too?

favorite place

what is your favorite place in the entire world?
mine is a bookshop.

any bookshop.
i'm not picky.

better yet –
with a door that chimes
a cheerful chirp
welcoming you in.

in a bookshop
you're immediately hit with
silence.
no sound
but the collective hum
of busy bee brains
immersed in fiction
weaving through rows
their fingers gingerly brushing over
perfect spines of paperbacks
opening their covers
subtly taking a sniff —
the smell cedar and cinnamon.

oh, how i wish they'd bottle that smell up
so on the gloomiest days
when the to-do list grows
and the babies are screaming
and my mind is reeling
and my skin is crawling
all i had to do was inhale
and be transported
to my favorite place.

seasons (growth)

seasons

'it's just a season,'
she says
as she rocks her newborn
in the middle of the night.

'it's just a season,'
she says
as she looks in the mirror
now embarrassed at the body
she recently considered beautiful.

'it's just a season,'
she says
to the dreary march new england sky
waiting for the flowers to bloom
and hoping that she will too.

snow

it snowed the first morning with you in our home.
i don't think you'll remember
but i will.

i brought you to your nursery window
and showed you fluffiness falling from the sky
           a homecoming gift.

snow makes me sentimental.
always has.

i'm in awe of how it can
control sound
manipulate the air
and make the world quiet
and loud
all at once.
a poet in its softest form.

snow stops time.

it personifies beauty.

and i can't thank snow enough
for helping me welcome
the most precious thing
i've ever held.
a tiny snowflake
made with love and teardrops and magic.
quiet and loud –
the greatest gift.

not my best

one day
i'd love for someone to say:
'that wasn't her best,'
because that means
something that i created
was their favorite.

winter babies

both my babies were born in early february
and it snowed every day until march.

i would sit on the couch
a new babe in my arms
and stare at the falling snow
with hatred in my eyes.

the snow and i are usually friends
but when you haven't left your house in over a month
i guess you start to hate the things you love …

      like yourself.

new england winters are always miserable.

they're dark
they're unbearable
    wet
they're agonizingly long
    dreary
      inconsistent

and they are never tired.

every bone in your body aches
from the cold
and from the long hours
sitting with a sleeping baby.

so, we wait patiently for spring
me and my winter baby.
and hope that when the sun wakes,
i can join the buds
and poke my head from the cold, hard earth
and start anew.

morning dew

the morning dew
sits on top of the lady mantle
fat, wet droplets
that shine
like crystals in a cave
waiting for the brightest star
to drink them up
and bring them home.

on a path less traveled

one morning i decided to go for a walk
on a path less traveled.

i stepped around jagged stones
and ducked under wayward branches
my sneakers squelching under fresh mud
following a trail to the unknown.

at first
i jumped at every sound.
a twig snapping
a bush rustling
a creature chattering
afraid that i would get snatched up
punished for wandering
for testing my
                limits.

but soon enough, those sounds
became familiar
and the voices in my head turned
from trepidation to praise.
and the brush cleared
and the mud dried
and i trusted my feet
to steer me back home.

growth

i will never tire of
planting seeds
and watching them grow
knowing they will return next spring
even stronger.

storm

as the storm rolls in
on this hot summer day
i wait in
        anticipation
rocking on my front porch
looking to the sky.

i watch as the clouds roll in
dark greys and blues
and listen as the percussion of the clouds
rumble toward me.

and the birds
once a chorus in the trees
fall to a hush
as they seek shelter
and bury their heads
in their feathery wings.

the air
once hazy and thick
and sweet like honey
stills.

and the trees start to applaud
as the wind sweeps through their branches
and they prepare for a nice, cold drink.

there's just something about soil

that makes me plunge my arms right in
straight up to my elbows
my fingers tickling worms
brushing roots
thumbing over stones
the sun warm on the back of my neck.

my arms are cold
from the earth's caress
and i am grounded
from its steady embrace
as i turn old into new
and wait for the seeds to bloom.

what makes a poet?

what makes a poet, really?
i pondered this the other day.

do we have to be broken?
a little
         disjointed?
unseen?

are all artists just chipped
fragmented?
using art to hold ourselves together?
to try to make us whole?

and if it weren't for that
song
painting
photograph
short story
sculpture
book
poem

would we just crack?

spring

there is something about spring
that i never noticed
until i moved in my home.

i've always wanted to fast-forward to summer
to watermelon and shade.
but what about the lungwort's leaves
stubbornly pushing through the cold ground
in early april?

or the smell of freshly mowed grass?
of warm mint from the garden that tingles your nose?
or the feeling of soil falling through your bare hands?

and what about the chilly mornings
that welcome warmer days?
or the dew sitting on leaves
waiting for the roots
to sip them up
so that the earth
can begin again?

lilac whispers

when i need a minute to clear my head
i go to my lilac tree
with its deep purple flowers
vibrant against the overcast sky
and its mighty branches
swaying tall
confidently
in the breeze
its paired blooms brushing shoulders
as if they are in on their own little secret.

is the secret
i wonder
that even on days when all seems
unbearable
unreasonable
unmanageable
beauty still exists?
tucked away
in my front yard
waiting for the right ears
to come along
lean in
and hear their whispers?

sunshine

what does sunshine taste like to you?
i taste strawberry lemonade
with a hint of lime.

oh – and mint
i taste that too.

sometimes when i write

my mind starts to scream.
… or does it buzz?

either way
the adrenaline takes hold
and my only function on this earth is to
create create create.

not just humans –
but *art*.

i sit propped up in my bed
with my notebook and my pen
scribbling until my back aches
until my hand cramps
and the only sounds
are my hand gliding over silky paper
and my husband's soft breathing
and my newborn's silent sighs
and a black cat's rhythmic purrs.

and i've never felt so present
during those moments where my mind is elsewhere.
scheming new ideas
plotting big dreams.

this is when i feel the most myself.

no cautionary thoughts
or perfectionist jabs.

just me sitting there
being
feeling
existing

create create create.

when springtime comes

i am five again
running through my yard
squealing at the buds
cheering them on
as they poke their sleepy heads
from the still-cold ground
ready for their second chance.

i read an anne bradstreet poem in college
where she talks about envying the spring
she acknowledges, in awe
that the trees have a chance for rejuvenation
the flower's encore
life begets life.

i understand her envy now.

nature always gets
that time for regrowth
but what about us?

and then i remember the new england winters
my tear-stained cheeks
hugging my knees
wishing for sun and warmth
waiting.

bradstreet and i are alike in many ways.
mothers
scared of winter
poets who write in the soft light among snoring creatures
our pens scratching paper
our minds unable to unrest.

we wish that we too can rise
from the dusty soil
squinting in the sunlight
ready to stretch our roots.

i understand her revelation now.
spring also exists for you and me
to brush the wet, cold snow off our shoulders
to turn our faces to the sun
and drink, drink, drink.
we can all start anew.

to the lilacs

goodbye to the lilacs
to their fragrant petals
and rich, purple blooms.
you are my favorite part of spring
with your rebellious flowers
that once screamed vividly
dangerously
against the overcast sky.

full

one afternoon
on a baby-free day
i grabbed my notebook
and went to the deck.

while i was sitting there
ice clinking in my glass
the birds told me the most amusing story
about crisp, cool mornings
that turn into warm, spring days
and how the sun
now bright
dries the dewy leaves on the trees
and kisses your skin
leaving you feeling warm and whole.

and then the birds laughed
as the light tickled their feathers
while a breeze rocked their nests
and they clung on the branches with their taloned feet.

and a rustle of leaves
applauded the birds' tale
and the entrance of a new season.

then started
the hum of motors
children laughing
and once again
the birds picked up their song
leaving my heart
and my notebook page
full.

summer

oh, sticky summer
with your warm, sweet air
that hits me right in the face
once i step outside.

and those gnats
that swarm right to my sweaty neck
making mad dashes
for my nose
that i furiously swat away
as i skulk down the driveway
to get the mail.

oh, summer, i won't miss your angry heat
once the leaves change
and the crisp breeze
dances through my hair.

but come winter
i know i will long
for your blistering rays.
i will long
for the crashing of blue-bodied waves.
and i will anxiously wait
for my sticky, new england summer
to come back again.

these days

i only have an appetite for stories and
 words
  that mean something.

sun

sneaking kisses
on soft, sun-screened skin
the smell of sweet coconut
all over.

'this is july,'
i think to myself
as my daughter picks clovers in the grass.

'mama!' she says,
holding out the most perfect gift.

rhode island

don't tell me that the beach
isn't one of your favorite places
in the world.

with its salty air
and its calling gulls
looking for a fallen chip
or a fish to eat
circling the rippling water
that sparkles in the sun.

with the ocean's tumbling waves
that crash against the shore
returning to its source
ready for its second chance
and third.
and fourth.

and fifth.

and oh, the sound they make!
a loud hush that calms my nerves
and caresses my sun-kissed, freckly skin.

the ocean reminds me
that i too can come back to the shore
plant my feet like an anchor in the gritty sand
and feel solace in the ebb and flow.

september

september is the beginning
of starting anew.

the time
to rip out messy pages
from a tattered notebook
its slate now clean
just waiting to be refilled.

and what about the maple trees?
do they feel the same
as they drop their leaves
feeling the heavy weight
fall from their branches?

are the trees also ready for something new?

when the sun rises in napa

when the sun rises in napa
it pauses.
it hides behind the clouds
using the misty air as a shield

and it waits.

the hares poke their heads
from their dusty burrows
and hop along the grapevines
their ears raised
alert
waiting.

the deer graze the fields
and the birds fly overhead
their circles breaking through the mist
and they wait.

the bees bumble by
drinking the flowers
filling their tiny bee bellies
sending vibrations in the
still air
and we all wait.

we all wait for the golden sun to
              break
through the clouds
and kiss the vines
and the hare's long ears
and the deer's soft head
and the bird's feathery wings
and the bee's furry belly
and my tired, freckled face
and welcome us to another day.

november

november came
like a frosty thief in the night
stealing our breath
turning our fingertips
ice cold.
our booted feet
crunching in the frozen leaves
watching as the sun slips
behind the heavy clouds
rubbing its sleepy eyes
and promising that it will return all the brighter.

through her eyes

there is nothing more beautiful
than witnessing the magic of christmas
through her eyes
                for the first time.

the poem

i guess i'm still waiting
for that poem.

for *the* poem

that will change our lives.

the poem that the publishers will take.

i guess i'm still waiting
for that 'aha! moment' to come.
where the words just fly across the page
the ink staining my fingers
as my mind creates magic.

i continue to read other poets
i soak in their genius
wondering what i am missing.

i feel the unspoken words in my chest.
they lie dormant like orphans
waiting for an author to give them a home.

am i just a fraud
wasting ink
and battery power
and canva templates?
are people just reading my dribble
just biding their time
as they wait
for some other poet
to write
the poem?

bones

i feel the winter chill pierce my bones
embedding its ugly head
deep in my marrow
i shudder in the unforgiving sunlight
gasping for warmth
wishing
waiting
begging
for spring.

the stream

i would walk down to the stream
when they were at their very worst.
they wouldn't even notice me slip out
barefoot –
just a small girl looking for some quiet.

a rock was placed there just for me
i believed.
contoured perfectly
to fit an eight-year-old's frame.
a tiny girl who would sit at the stream,
her arms hugging her knees,
waiting for the silence to come.

she would listen to the crickets
and sing their familiar tune
and the frogs would join in
because they knew it too.

and she'd close her eyes
and picture her favorite place
and wish
that one day
that place
would become her home.

daffodils

yellow daffodils
on a cloudy day
gives me hope.

the hummingbird

i was sitting on my deck
embracing the sun's sweet kisses
when out of the corner of my eye
i saw a hummingbird land in my garden.

'don't breathe, don't move,'
i thought
as i took in this tiny-winged creature
its body so small
but with an even larger presence.

i watched as it flitted toward
the planter filled with honeybells
and with its body mid air
i heard a slight buzz
and i watched it take a drink.
big gulps.
it hopped from bell to bell
creating its own nectarean melody.

and once it took its fill
it left as fast as it came.

and i thought to myself:
'how lucky are we
to live in a world
where beauty like that exists?'

acknowledgments

to my husband: you are a true gift. your steadfast support and encouragement made this possible. thank you for always pushing me to sit out on the deck with my pink notebook.

to my girls: you are light. you are messy and sweet and fun. there is a lot of sadness in here, but just know that i wouldn't change this life for the world.
you are everything i wished for.

to cecilia gigliotti: thank you for your keen eyes, encouraging nudges, and pep talks all the way from germany. anyway, the wind blows …

to my best friend, nicki: thank you for your friendship. i'm sorry my poems keep making you cry.

to hannah hawthorne: thank you for helping make this book beautiful with your talent and guidance.

to my classy classic ladies, to my rolling mama group chats, to my bookstagram community, my friends, my family: my goodness. you really know how to make a girl feel loved and seen. i was never nervous to post my work for i knew you had my back. i am eternally grateful for this support system that spans across every corner of the world.

and to those who have this book in your hands (in any format): thank you. i hope these poems reach you in some way. i hope they help you feel less alone. be well.

about the author

kassondra mangione lives in connecticut with her husband, two daughters, three cats, and many, many bookshelves. She grew up on the connecticut shoreline with a love of writing, music, and theatre. kassondra earned a bachelor's degree in journalism and a master's degree in english. she is the host of the podcast, "grace & grit: navigating postpartum & parenthood," where mothers and parents share their pregnancy, postpartum, and motherhood journeys.
her podcast was inspired by her poems, which she started writing in april 2022.

kassondra loves coffee, gardening, her peloton bike, and scribbling in her notebooks.
this is her first self-published work.

find her online:
www.keepitkassual.com
@keepitkassual
@graceandgrit_podcast

Printed in the USA
CPSIA information can be obtained
at www.ICGtesting.com
CBHW071441080824
12890CB00008B/384